NOOM I
GUIDE C

Learn the Science to Losing Weight, Restoring Metabolism & Rebuilding Your Health with Complete Food List Meal Plan & Healthy Recipes.

Lois Adams

Copyright © 2023–

Lois Adams

ISBN:

Printed in the United States of America

Disclaimer
This publication is designed to provide competent and reliable information regarding the subject covered. However, the views expressed in this publication are those of the author alone, and should not be taken as expert instruction or professional advice. The reader is responsible for his or her actions. The author hereby disclaims any responsibility or liability whatsoever that is incurred from the use or application of the contents of this publication by the purchaser of the reader. The purchaser or reader is hereby responsible for his or her actions.

All rights reserved. No part of this publication may be reproduced, distributed, or transmitted in any form or by any means, including photocopying, recording, or other electronic or mechanical methods, without the prior written permission of the publisher, except in the case of brief quotations embodied in critical reviews and certain other non-commercial uses permitted by copyright law. For permission requests, write to the publisher, addressed at the address below

TABLE OF CONTENTS

Introduction 6

CHAPTER ONE 8

the noom diet 8

   What is Noom Diet? 8

   How the Noom Diet works 10

   Benefits of Noom Diet 14

CHAPTER TWO 19

Noom Diet Food List 19

   Green Foods 19

   Whole Grains 25

   Yellow foods 29

   Red Foods 38

Chapter three 45

NOOM DIET SHOPPING LIST 45

   Breakfast Shopping List 45

Lunch Shopping List 48

Dinner Shopping List 50

Snack Shopping List 52

chapter four 54

Noom Diet Meal Plans 54

21 Day Breakfast Meal Plan 54

21-Day Lunch Meal Plan 59

Dinner Meal Plan 64

21-Day Snack Meal Plan 70

CHAPTER FIVE 75

RECIPES FOR NOOM DIET FOOD LIST 75

Green Foods Recipes 75

Yellow Foods Recipes 93

Red Foods Recipes 107

CHAPTER SIX 127

Noom Diet Tips and Tricks 127

How to stay on track with Noom Diet. 127

How to make Healthy Food Choices . 129

How to Plan your Meals and Snacks . 132

How to Deal with Cravings.................. 134

CONCLUSION 137

INTRODUCTION

The Noom Diet is a well-liked weight loss plan that encourages participants to develop lifelong patterns of healthful behavior. The food list is central to the Noom Diet, which emphasizes natural, nutrient-dense meals while reducing the intake of processed and high-calorie options. In encouraging a healthy, well-rounded diet, this strategy aims to aid in weight loss and general wellness.

The Noom Diet food list contains a diverse selection of items from many dietary groups, such as vegetables and fruits, whole grains, lean meats, including healthy fats. This strategy guarantees that dieters take in a wide range of vitamins, and minerals, including antioxidants, all of which are necessary for good health.

The Noom Diet does more than just tell you what to eat; it also tells you how much to consume and stresses the need of being conscious about food choices. The Noom Diet seeks to induce lasting changes in one's behavior that will allow for long-term success in weight reduction by fostering a more nuanced knowledge of one's connection with food as well as the body.

CHAPTER ONE

THE NOOM DIET

What is Noom Diet?

The well-known Noom Diet uses technology, psychology-based behavior modification strategies, and individualized coaching to assist users in reaching their weight reduction objectives. The service gives customers access to individualized diet plans, fitness schedules, and support from a specialized coach using a mobile app as well as a virtual coaching system.

Instead, then emphasizing dietary restriction, the Noom Diet promotes wholesome eating practices and long-lasting lifestyle modifications. The software classifies meals according to their calorie density and gives each category a color, with greens being the category with the greatest nutrients, then yellow, and eventually red.

When it comes to the mental blocks that prevent people from losing weight, the Noom Diet takes a behavioral modification approach. To assist users to recognize and alter bad eating patterns, the software provides daily articles, and quizzes, including interactive challenges. The Noom Diet software also provides tools for users to keep tabs on their weight, physical activity, and meals, as well as a support network where they can interact and discuss their success. After the program's free trial, users can pick and choose whether to stick with a premium membership.

The Noom Diet approach, in general, is designed to serve as a long-term weight reduction strategy that emphasizes establishing durable adjustments to food and activity habits rather than depending on brief diets or fast fixes.

How the Noom Diet works

Popular weight reduction program The Noom Diet employs a tailored strategy to assist people to achieve their weight loss objectives. Here is how it works:

Alteration of Behavior:

Noom focuses on changing habits linked to diet, exercise, and self-care. They provide daily activities and challenges to assist you in developing healthy habits which can result in long-term weight reduction success.

Calorie Counting:

Noom has a color-coded approach to assist you in tracking your daily calorie consumption. Depending on their calorie density, meals are classified as green, yellow, or red, with green foods becoming the least dense as well as red foods being the densest.

Coaching that is Tailored to the Individual:

Users of Noom get a one-on-one coach who gives support and direction during the weight reduction process. They assist users in setting realistic objectives while also providing accountability and inspiration to maintain their momentum.

Group Assistance:

Noom members get access to a group of other people who are also attempting to lose weight. This group offers members encouragement and assistance to help them remain on track.

Education:

Noom teaches users about healthy eating practices, and portion control, including mindful eating. They also offer advice on how to eat healthily and incorporate a workout into everyday activities.

Psychological Behavior:

Noom employs behavioral psychology concepts to assist users in changing their eating and exercise habits and behaviors. They emphasize the need of cultivating a growth mindset, foster self-reflection including self-awareness, and offer positive reinforcement.

System of Color Coding:

Noom categorizes foods based on calorie density using a color-coding method. Green foods are nutrient-dense and low in calories, whereas red foods have high in calories and must be taken in moderation.

Unique meal Plans:

Noom creates customized meal plans for consumers based on their dietary choices, health objectives, and lifestyle. The meal plans offer a wide range of nutritious and healthy meals that are simple to prepare and appropriate for various meal times and circumstances.

Tracking Your Fitness:

By measuring users' activity levels via the app, Noom encourages them to include exercise in their everyday routines. Users may establish objectives, measure their progress, then receive support and encouragement from their coach as well as the group.

Accountability and Assistance:

Users of Noom get a dedicated coach who gives support and direction during the weight reduction process. Users may also interact with a group of other users that are also attempting to lose weight. This accountability and support can help people stay inspired as well as on track toward their goals.

Benefits of Noom Diet

Noom is a popular weight loss and diet reduction program that uses a mobile app and individualized coaching to assist individuals in developing healthy habits and losing weight. These are a few benefits of the Noom diet:

Individualized Coaching:

The Noom team consists of certified nutritionists, and behavioral psychologists, including personal trainers that provide individualized coaching. This coaching is meant to help you create goals, maintain accountability, and make lasting changes to your lifestyle and eating habits.

Emphasis on Healthful Practices:

Noom focuses on creating healthy behaviors rather than calorie tracking or dietary restriction.

This method can help you establish a healthy connection with food and prevent the yo-yo dieting cycle.

Flexible and Sustainable:

Noom is a flexible diet plan that allows you to consume a range of meals and does not need you to completely abstain from your favorite foods. This makes it simpler to adhere to over the long run and can help you achieve sustainable weight reduction.

Behavior Modification:

Noom employs behavioral modification strategies, such as setting modest, attainable objectives and recognizing your victories along the way, to help you build better habits. This can help you maintain motivation and increase your confidence in your capacity to make great changes.

Beneficial Community:

You may interact with other members, discuss your triumphs and problems, and receive support from coaches and other members through Noom's online community.

Evidence-Based Strategy:

The Noom method is founded on the most recent research in nutrition, psychology, as well as behavior modification. This evidence-based strategy can help you make educated health and well-being decisions.

Education and Understanding:

Noom offers nutrition, portion sizes, and good eating practices instruction. This information may help you make intelligent choices about what you eat and why, as well as increase your knowledge of how to stay at an appropriate weight.

Monitoring and Responsibility:

The Noom app lets you track your food consumption, physical activity, and weight reduction progress. This monitoring can help you remain accountable for your objectives and encourage you to keep making progress.

Individualized Food Plans:

Noom offers personalized meal plans that are suited to your interests, lifestyle, and objectives. This might help you make better food selections and reduce meal planning stress.

Emphasis on Self-Care:

Noom promotes the need for self-care, including enough sleep, stress management, and mental health treatment. This comprehensive approach to well-being can help you accomplish not only weight reduction but also general health and well-being.

No Dietary Limitations:

Noom does not exclude particular foods or dietary groups, unlike other diets. Instead, it promotes moderation and portion management, which can aid in the development of a better relationship with food.

Positive Reinforcement:

Noom emphasizes positive reinforcement, praising your accomplishments and boosting your confidence in your capacity to make good decisions. This might help you maintain your motivation and commitment to your weight reduction objectives.

CHAPTER TWO

NOOM DIET FOOD LIST

Green Foods

Vegetables

The term "green foods" refers to those that are abundant in nutrients like vitamins, minerals, and some other nutrients. Many leafy greens may be included on the Noom diet's approved food list.

Users of the well-known weight-loss program Noom are urged to eat healthily in a sustainable manner. Vegetables have several beneficial properties, including being low in fat and rich in fiber. Vegetables that are typical in a Noom proper diet plan include the following:

The Leafy Greens:

Greens like spinach, kale, as well as lettuce, are packed with nutrients like vitamin supplements A, C, K, and folate, not to mention fiber and antioxidants.

Vegetables with Cruciform Crucifixes:

Broccoli, cauliflower, cabbage, with Brussels sprouts are all examples of cruciferous vegetables. These plants are rich in fiber, vitamins C and K, including antioxidants. In addition, they contain a lot of plant-based protein.

Trussed Roots:

Allium vegetables like carrots, beets, turnips, as well as sweet potatoes are excellent sources of fiber, vitamins C and A, and minerals like potassium and magnesium.

Veggies in the Nightshade Family:

Tomatoes, peppers, plus eggplant all belong to the nightshade family of vegetables, which are high in antioxidants and vitamins A and C. In addition, they have the chemical capsaicin, which has been shown to increase metabolic rate and facilitate weight loss.

Vegetable Onions:

Garlic, onions, and leeks are all members of the allium plant family, which is known for its high levels of antioxidants and sulfur-containing compounds that have been shown to reduce inflammation and strengthen the immune system.

Pumpkins and Winter Squash:

The fiber, vitamins A and C, as well as the potassium content of squashes and gourds, is very high.

Leguminous:

All three of these legumes—beans, lentils, and chickpeas—are highly nutritious.

Mushrooms:

Mushrooms have few calories, but plenty of fiber and healthy compounds called antioxidants. B vitamins as well as minerals like selenium are also present.

Sea Vegetables:

Nori, kelp, with wakame, are all types of sea vegetables that are high in iodine, a mineral necessary for healthy thyroid function. They are also a good source of fiber, vitamins, plus minerals.

Sprouts:

Alfalfa, broccoli, as well as mung bean sprouts, are just a few examples of the many kinds of sprouts that may be found and eaten for their high nutrient and enzyme content.

Fruits

A plant-based, whole-food diet is at the heart of the Noom weight loss regimen. Fruits are included in plentiful quantities on the Noom diet food list.

Find out more about the Noom diet-approved fruits below.

Berries:

Berries are an excellent supplier of fiber, vitamins, including antioxidants. Berries come in a wide variety, but some common ones are strawberries, blueberries, raspberries, and blackberries, among cranberry.

Fruits that contain citric acid:

Vitamin C, fiber, and other plant chemicals that are good for you may be found in abundance in citrus fruits. Citrus fruits involve oranges, grapefruits, lemons, limes, as well as tangerines, just to name a few.

Hard-Skinned Fruits:

Juicy and delicious, stone fruits are characterized by a central pit or stone. Stone fruits are a kind of fruit that includes things like plums, apricots, cherries, and peaches.

Tropical fruits:

Vitamins, minerals, plus antioxidants abound in many tropical fruits. Mangoes, pineapples, bananas, papayas, and guavas are all examples of tropical fruits.

Apples and pears:

Pears and apples would both be high in fiber and low in calories, offering them a wonderful snack option. They also include vitamins, minerals, and even antioxidants.

Melons:

Because of their high water content and low-calorie count, melons are a healthy and delicious way to stay hydrated. Fruits like watermelon, cantaloupe, as well as honeydew, are all examples of melons.

Grapes:

Grapes have antioxidants and are rich in vitamins and minerals. Red, green, as well as purple are just a few of the hues available.

Kiwi:

Low in fat and packed with fiber, Vitamin C, and potassium, kiwis are a healthy addition to any diet. Their flavor is sour, and they have fuzzy brown skin that must be peeled.

Whole Grains

There are various varieties of whole grains on the Noom Diet food list that you may incorporate into your meals. These whole grains are high in nutrients and can give long-lasting energy as well as other health advantages. Here are some specifics about the whole grains in the Noom Diet food list:

Rice, brown:

Both bran, germ, as well as endosperm, are all present in a serving of brown rice, making it a complete grain. It contains fiber, vitamins, plus minerals, and it can help manage blood sugar levels.

Quinoa:

Quinoa is a gluten-free, high-protein, fiber-rich whole grain. It's also high in vitamins and minerals including iron, magnesium, as well as zinc.

Oats:

Oats are high in fiber, protein, and minerals such as vitamin E plus magnesium. They can also aid in cholesterol reduction and heart health.

Barley:

Barley is a complete grain with a high fiber and protein content. It is also rich in minerals and vitamins like iron, magnesium, and zinc.

Buckwheat:

Buckwheat is a complete grain that is gluten-free and high in fiber, and protein, including minerals like magnesium as well as potassium. It also contains a lot of antioxidants.

Whole Wheat flour:

Whole wheat is high in fiber, protein, and minerals such as B vitamins and iron. It may also help reduce the risk of cardiovascular illnesses as well as type 2 diabetes.

Millet:

Millet is a gluten-free whole grain with a high fiber and protein content. It is also rich in minerals and vitamins like magnesium and phosphorus.

Lean proteins:

The Noom diet lacks a set list of "lean proteins," yet it does advocate for including a variety of different protein sources in meals. These are some lean protein sources that might be part of a Noom-friendly diet:

Chicken thigh:

Desiccated, boneless chicken breast is a high-protein food. A 3-ounce portion has around 25 grams of protein.

Chicken breast:

Turkey breast, like chicken breast, is low in fat and high in protein. A 3-ounce portion has around 26 grams of protein.

Fish:

Salmon, tuna, as well as tilapia are also all excellent sources of high-quality protein. A 3-ounce portion of salmon has around 22 grams of protein, whereas a 3-ounce dish of tuna has approximately 25 grams of protein.

Eggs:

Eggs are a great way to get your protein in, and they're OK on the Noom diet. A big egg has around six grams of protein per serving.

Yogurt from Greece:

Greek yogurt is a high-protein food that may be used as a foundation for smoothies as well as a snack. A 6-ounce portion has around 17 grams of protein.

Beans:

Plant-based protein may be found in beans such as black beans, chickpeas, among lentils. A 1/2 cup portion of black beans has around eight grams of protein.

Yellow foods

The Noom Health Food List consists of an assortment of color-coded items. Yellow foods are often connected with carbs, and consuming complete, raw foods from the yellow food category is encouraged. Consuming a range of yellow foods can assist satisfy energy demands by providing critical vitamins, minerals, and fiber. Yellow foods can also aid in maintaining stable blood sugar levels, boosting energy, and promoting satiety. include grains, starchy veggies, and some fruits.

Carbohydrate-Rich Veggies:

Starchy veggies are vegetables with a high starch and carbohydrate content. While they are an excellent source of energy, they contain more calories than non-starchy veggies. Noom is a method for weight loss that emphasizes a balanced, whole-food diet. Below are instances of starchy vegetables permitted on the Noom diet:

Potatoes:

This comprises all potato kinds including sweet potatoes, white potatoes, and red potatoes. Potatoes are a rich source of carbs, as well as fiber, vitamin C, and potassium.

Corn:

Corn is a starchy food rich in fiber, vitamin C, as well as thiamin. Fresh corn on the cob is a favorite summertime vegetable, but it is frequently available in canned or frozen form.

Squash:

This comprises spaghetti squash, butternut squash, and acorn squash. The vegetable squash is rich in fiber, vitamin A, plus potassium.

Peas:

Peas are starchy, high-protein, high-fiber, and vitamin A and C-rich vegetables. They are frequently available frozen and may be used in soups, stews, and side dishes.

Beets:

Beets are a root vegetable that is strong in carbs, as well as an excellent source of fiber, folate, and manganese. They are most often roasted or boiled before being served in salads or as an additional side dish.

Yams:

Yams are a carbohydrate vegetable that resembles sweet potatoes but is typically bigger and has a coarser skin. They are rich in dietary fiber, potassium, with vitamin C.

Plantains:

Similar to bananas, plantains are however a starchy vegetable that would be normally prepared before consumption. They are commonly used in the cuisines of Latin America and the Caribbean and may be consumed fried, baked, or even boiled.

Dairy Products

Noom is a popular rapid weight loss program that emphasizes the development of good habits and the implementation of lasting lifestyle modifications. The Noom diet stresses entire, nutrient-dense foods, particularly dairy products, in its food list. Here are some specifics regarding the dairy products which are permitted on the Noom diet:

Skim milk:

Skim milk is an excellent alternative for calcium, vitamin D, as well as protein, but it is lower in calories and fat than full milk.

Greek yogurt:

Greek yogurt is a low-fat, high-protein dairy product that can be substituted for sour cream, cream cheese, and mayonnaise. Opt for Greek yogurt that is basic and unsweetened to avoid extra sugars.

Cottage cheese:

Cottage cheese is an excellent source of protein plus calcium, and it has a low caloric content. Nevertheless, it can be heavy in salt, so search for kinds that are reduced in sodium.

Reduced-calorie cheese:

Reduced-fat cheese provides calcium as well as protein, but less fat and fewer calories than regular cheese. Search for options that are low in salt and do not contain additional sweeteners.

Almond milk:

Almond milk is a low-calorie and low-fat non-dairy alternative to milk. It is not, however, a good supplier of protein and calcium, thus it should not be substituted for dairy products.

Legumes

Legumes are an excellent plant-based source of protein, fiber, and some other necessary elements. They are an essential component of a nutritious and well-balanced diet, such as the Noom diet. Common legumes that could be included in a Noom diet plan include as follows.

Chickpeas:

Chickpeas are a popular legume that is high in protein, fiber, plus iron. They are also referred to as garbanzo beans. They may very well be utilized in several recipes, including hummus, salads, and even soups.

Lentils:

Lentils are a kind of legume that is available in brown, green, as well as red hues. They are an excellent source of protein, and fiber, with complex carbs, and may be utilized in soups, stews, and salads, as well as a substitute for meat in burgers and other foods.

Beans, black:

Black beans are an excellent source of protein, fiber, iron, plus antioxidants. In Latin American cuisine, they are often used in soups, salads, and as fillings for burritos and tacos.

Renny beans:

Kidney beans are an adaptable legume that may be utilized in soups, salads, and chili. They contain ample amounts of protein, fiber, iron, plus folate.

Peas:

Peas are a kind of legume that is rich in dietary fiber, protein, and other vitamins and minerals. They may be included in salads, soups, and side dishes.

Soybeans:

Soybeans are a high-protein legume extensively employed in the production of tofu, soy milk, and some other soy-based goods. They are also utilized in Asian cuisine, where they may be included in stir-fries, soups, and salads.

Oils and Fats

The Noom Diet food list classifies foods according to their caloric density as well as nutritional value, and hence includes a range of fats and oils in moderation. Below are some of the fats and oils that are permitted on the Noom Diet:

Seeds and Nuts:

Nuts and seeds, including almonds, cashews, and even sunflower seeds, are excellent sources of protein and healthy fats. They are extremely heavy in calories, thus moderation is required while consuming them.

Avocado:

Avocado is rich in monounsaturated fats, fiber, and potassium. It may be substituted for mayonnaise or butter in a variety of recipes, including salad dressings, smoothies, and spreads.

Olive Oil:

Olive oil is a monounsaturated fatty acid-rich, heart-healthy fat. It is used often in cooking including salad dressings.

Coconut Oil:

Research shows that coconut oil may have health advantages despite its high saturated fat content. It is utilized frequently in both baking and cooking.

Flaxseed Oil:

Omega-3 fatty acids are essential to heart health, and flaxseed oil is a rich source of them. It may be included in salad dressings and smoothies.

Red Foods

Foods rich in antioxidants, vitamins, minerals, and fiber are commonplace on Noom Diet Food Lists, which are often presented in a red color scheme. Apples, beets, cherries, cranberries, berries, raspberries, red peppers, tomatoes, plus red onions are only some examples of red foods. All of these options are nutrient-rich, low in calories, as well as good for your health in many ways, including lowering inflammation, easing digestive issues, and bolstering your immune system. Some kinds of cancer may be prevented by eating more red foods, which have been shown to have anti-cancer qualities. Consuming a diverse range of red foods is an excellent strategy for obtaining the nutrients you need and keeping your weight in check.

Processed Foods

Foods that have been changed from their original form, often for better flavor, texture, or preservation, are classified as processed. The following are some common processed foods:

Snacks in a box:

Snack foods such as chips, crackers, granola bars, and the like tend to be loaded with empty calories, sodium, and bad fats.

Quick meals:

Fast food like burgers, fries, and pizza can be rich in salt, saturated fat, and calories.

Beverages laden with sugar:

Weight gain as well as other health issues have been linked to the consumption of sugary beverages including soda, energy drinks, and especially sports drinks.

Dishes that can be cooked from frozen:

Sodium, preservatives, and bad fats tend to be more abundant in frozen meals and main dishes.

Meals from a can:

Sugar, salt, and preservatives are sometimes added to canned soups, veggies, and fruits.

High Calories Foods:

Nuts and nut kinds of butter - Nuts contain a lot of calories, but they're also heavy in fiber, protein, and healthy fats that can keep you feeling full for longer. A healthy diet may contain nuts and nut butter, but it's crucial to pay attention to portion quantities.

Avocados are an excellent complement to meals since they are packed with fiber, heart-healthy monounsaturated fats, and other minerals. As a result of their high-calorie content, it's crucial to eat them in moderation.

Cheese is a high-calorie item that can be included in a balanced diet in moderation. It contains a lot of saturated fat but also a lot of protein, calcium, and other minerals.

Dark chocolate has a lot of antioxidants and some other healthy elements, but it's also quite calorie-dense. It's great to indulge sometimes rather than regularly.

Whole grains - Whole grains include more calories than refined grains, but they are also more nutrient-dense and can help you feel full for longer. Examples of whole grains include quinoa, brown rice, and even whole pasta. Keeping an eye on portion sizes and balancing them with other lower-calorie items is crucial.

Sweets and Desserts

- Cake - According to the Noom diet, most cakes are red foods since they are heavy in calories, sugar, and fat.
- Cookies are often baked with flour, sugar, and butter, which gives them a high calorie and fat content.
- Candy - According to the Noom diet, the majority of sweets are red foods since they are heavy in calories and sugar.
- Ice cream is a red item on the Noom diet because it is heavy in calories, sugar, as well as fat.
- Chocolate - While milk chocolate and other varieties of chocolate candies are often heavy in sugar and calories and are categorized as red foods in the Noom diet, dark chocolate may be a nutritious pleasure when consumed in moderation.

- Pastries are considered red foods in the Noom diet since they often include a lot of calories and fat, including croissants, Danishes, and muffins.

High-Fat Foods:

Deep-fried dishes including fries, fried chicken, onion rings, and even tempura are included in the category of fried foods.

High-fat cuts of beef, and hog, including lamb, such as ribeye steak, prime rib, bacon, and sausage, especially lamb chops, are included in the category of fatty meats.

Whole milk, full-fat cheese, butter, cream, and even ice cream are all examples of full-fat dairy products.

Processed meats - This category includes sausage, hot dogs, bacon, and deli meats.

Fast food consists of fried chicken sandwiches, cheeseburgers, hamburgers, and pizza.

CHAPTER THREE

NOOM DIET SHOPPING LIST

Breakfast Shopping List

The Noom diet emphasizes eating full, nutrient-dense meals while minimizing processed and high-calorie items. Breakfast options that would be good for the Noom diet include:

- ❖ Fresh fruit: Select fiber-rich, low-sugar fruits such as berries, apples, pears, and especially citrus fruits.
- ❖ Greek yogurt is high in protein and calcium and may be mixed with fresh fruit, nuts, and mixed seeds for extra taste and texture.
- ❖ Cereals and oatmeal produced from whole grains and with a minimal amount of added sugar are good options. For extra taste and texture, add fresh fruit and nuts.

- ❖ Eggs: Eggs are a high-protein food that may be served in a variety of ways, including scrambled, boiled, or baked.
- ❖ Try to choose slices of bread that are high in fiber and have little to no added sugar, such as an English muffin or toast prepared with whole grains. To add taste and nutrition, top either avocado, nut butter, or low-fat cheese.
- ❖ Smoothies: For a nutrient-dense breakfast on the run, combine fresh or frozen fruits, Greek yogurt, as well as a drink of your choosing (such as almond milk or coconut water).
- ❖ Vegetables: Including veggies in your breakfast is an excellent method to increase your daily fiber and vitamin consumption. To your morning bowl or omelet, try sautéed spinach, and sliced tomatoes, with roasted sweet potatoes.
- ❖ Foods high in good fats, protein, and fiber, including nuts and seeds, are

important for a balanced diet. To add crunch and nutrients to your cereal or yogurt, sprinkle with chopped almonds, walnut, or chia seeds.

- ❖ Low-fat dairy: Aside from Greek yogurt, low-fat milk, as well as cheese, can be included in a nutritious breakfast. Seek skim or 1% milk, as well as low-fat and low-sodium cheeses.
- ❖ Whole-grain pancakes or waffles: On the Noom diet, you may still have pancakes and waffles as long as you pick whole-grain types and restrict added sweets. To add sweetness, top with fresh fruit and a drizzle of honey or maple syrup.
- ❖ Breakfast burrito or wrap: Layer scrambled eggs, black beans, salsa, and avocado over a whole-grain tortilla for a substantial and tasty breakfast high in protein and fiber.
- ❖ Look for foods that are minimally processed, reduced in added sugars and

salt, and high in nutrients such as fiber, protein, including healthy fats when shopping for breakfast products on the Noom diet. Remember to watch your portion sizes and eat consciously, paying attention to your hunger or fullness cues.

Lunch Shopping List

The Noom diet prioritizes complete, nutrient-dense, low-calorie meals that are high in fiber as well as protein. Here are a few food things you may want to consider buying for your lunch:

- ❖ Lean proteins: Fish, tofu, legumes, lentils, chicken, turkey, poultry, and low-fat milk products are all great protein sources that may make you feel content and full.
- ❖ Vegetables: Add bulk as well as nutrition to your meals without increasing the calorie count by choosing non-starchy veggies such as leafy greens, broccoli,

cauliflower, carrots, and even bell peppers.

- ❖ Fruits: Berries, apples, oranges, and bananas, among others, may provide natural sweetness and fiber to your meals. Fruits can also be consumed frozen or fresh.
- ❖ You can get the fiber and complex carbs you need to feel full from whole grains like quinoa, brown rice, whole wheat bread, and whole wheat pasta.
- ❖ Nuts, seeds, avocados, as well as olive oil are all good fat sources that may assist with feeling full and deliver necessary nutrients.

Dinner Shopping List

The Noom diet emphasizes whole foods and a nutritious diet as a way to lose weight in a healthy, long-term way. Consider adding the following food groups as well as items to your grocery list for a Noom-friendly dinner:

- ❖ Chicken breast, turkey breast, fish (like salmon, tuna, and cod), lean beef, tofu, tempeh, as well as legumes are all good sources of lean proteins (such as lentils, chickpeas, and black beans).
- ❖ Leafy greens like spinach, kale, arugula, broccoli, cauliflower, carrots, bell peppers, mushrooms, zucchini, or even asparagus are all non-starchy vegetables.
- ❖ Potatoes, yams, butternut squash, but also corn are all vegetables that are high in starch.

- ❖ Brown rice, quinoa, whole wheat pasta, and whole grain bread are all examples of whole grains.
- ❖ Avocado, nuts (like almonds as well as walnuts), seeds (like chia and flax), as well as olive oil are all good sources of healthy fats.

Additional Items:

Chicken breasts with no bones and no skin

New spinach

Broccoli florets

Sweet potatoes

The brown rice

Avocado

Avocado

Oil from olives

Snack Shopping List

The Noom diet recommends eating nutritious snacks between meals to prevent binge eating. Noom recommends picking snacks that are high in nutrients and have few calories. Here are some snack ideas to stock up on:

Raw fruits such as apples, bananas, oranges, berries, etc.

Sticks of raw vegetables like carrots, cucumber, bell pepper, etc.

Almonds, cashews, pistachios, and other tree nuts.

Plant seeds such as chia seeds, pumpkin seeds, chia seeds, etc.

Dairy products that are low in fat, such as Greek yogurt, cottage cheese, etc.

Munch on some nut butter as well as hummus with some rice cakes or whole-grain crackers.

Boiled eggs

popped corn with only air.

Dehydrated fruit (in moderation and without added sugars).

Substances are similar to dark chocolate (in moderation).

CHAPTER FOUR

NOOM DIET MEAL PLANS

21 Day Breakfast Meal Plan

Day 1: July 24

Greek yogurt containing blueberries as well as a garnish of chopped almonds, along with scrambled eggs, spinach, tomatoes, and bread made from whole grains

Day 2: July 25

Oats left in the fridge overnight with almond milk, chia seeds, banana slices, and a sprinkle of honey

a cooked egg and sliced turkey

Day 3: July 26

Vegetable omelet with peppers, onions, and mushrooms, over whole-grain bread.

piece of apple with almond butter

Day 4: July 27

Sliced peaches with cinnamon sprinkled over cottage cheese

cooked egg and turkey bacon

Day 5: July 28

Waffles made of whole grains served with berries and Greek yogurt.

A slice of fruit with a variety of nuts

Day 6: July 29

Poached egg, sliced tomatoes, and avocado toast

Strawberries in Greek yogurt with a dash of oats

Day 7: 30/7

Breakfast burrito on a whole-grain tortilla with scrambled eggs, black beans, and salsa.

orange slices

Day 8: 31/7

spinach, banana, almond butter, with peanut butter in a protein smoothie

turkey sausage with a hard-boiled egg

Day 9:

Using mashed bananas, eggs, and mixed oats to make the pancakes, they are then topped with Greek yogurt and berries.

A slice of fruit with a variety of nuts

Day 10:

Greek yogurt over sliced banana, honey, as well as a sprinkling of cinnamon

cooked egg and turkey bacon

Day 11:

Served with whole-grain bread and an egg white omelet with spinach as well as mushrooms.

piece of apple with almond butter

Day 12:

Sliced peaches with cinnamon sprinkled over cottage cheese

a cooked egg and turkey sausage

Day 13: 5/8

Breakfast sandwich with turkey bacon, scrambled eggs, and a whole-grain English muffin.

A slice of fruit with a variety of nuts

Day 14: 6/8

Almond milk, spinach, mixed berries, and protein powder in a protein smoothie

turkey sausage with a hard-boiled egg

Day 15: 7/8

Strawberries in Greek yogurt with a dash of oats

a cooked egg and sliced turkey

Day 16: 8/8

Turkey bacon, a cooked egg, and oatmeal with sliced apples, cinnamon, and chopped nuts

Day 17: 9|8

Vegetable omelet with peppers, onions, and mushrooms, over whole-grain bread.

A slice of fruit with a variety of nuts

Day 18: 10|8

Waffles made of whole grains served with berries and Greek yogurt.

a cooked egg and turkey sausage

Day 19: 11|8

Poached egg, sliced tomatoes, and avocado toast

piece of apple with almond butter

Day 20: 12|8

Blueberries in Greek yogurt with a sprinkling of chopped nuts

Turkey bacon and a hard-boiled egg

Day 21: 13/8

Breakfast burrito on a whole-grain tortilla containing poached eggs, black beans, plus salsa.

A slice of fruit with a variety of nuts

21-Day Lunch Meal Plan

Day 1: 24/7

Grilled chicken breast with cherry tomatoes and balsamic vinaigrette dressings over a bed of mixed greens

Sweet potato wedges, roasted

Day 2: 25/7

Tuna salad on whole-grain bread with light mayonnaise, diced celery, and onion.

Cucumber slices with hummus dip

Day 3: 26/7

Apple slices with almond butter grilled salmon with lemon and dill served with quinoa and steamed broccoli

Day 4: 27/7

Soup with black beans, chopped tomatoes, red peppers, and onions

Whole-grain roll, small

Day 5: 28/7

Grilled chicken and veggie kabobs served with brown rice and fresh fruit

Day 6: 29/7

Hummus, avocado, chopped carrots, and spinach wrapped in a whole-grain wrap

Ranch-dressed baby carrots

Day 7: 30/7

Grilled shrimp and veggie skewers with roasted asparagus on the side

Sliced pears with cottage cheese

Day 8: 31/7

Soup with lentils, carrots, celery, with onions

Crackers made from whole grains

Day 9: 1/8

Sandwich with turkey and cheese on whole-grain bread with lettuce and tomato

Tzatziki dip with sliced bell peppers

Day 10: 2/8

Caesar salad with grilled chicken, whole-grain croutons, and a mild Caesar dressing

Grapes

Day 11: 3/8

Broccoli, snow peas, carrots, and mushrooms are stir-fried with brown rice.

Clementine

Day 12: 4/8

Pesto-marinated grilled chicken breast served alongside roasted sweet potatoes with green beans

Almond butter with apple slices

Day 13: 5|8

Wrap of vegetables and hummus with avocado plus roasted red peppers

Ranch-dressed baby carrots

Day 14: 6|8

Chili with turkey, chopped tomatoes, and black beans

Whole-grain roll, small

Day 15: 7|8

Grilled shrimp and veggie skewers with roasted asparagus on the side

Sliced pears with cottage cheese

Day 16: 8/8

Orange slices with a spinach and feta omelet and whole-grain bread

Day 17: 9/8

Salad of quinoa and black beans with chopped bell peppers and red onion

Fresh berries on Greek yogurt

Day 18: 10/8

Grilled chicken breast with cherry tomatoes and balsamic vinaigrette dressing over a bed of mixed greens

Sweet potato wedges, roasted

Day 19: 11/8

Tuna salad on whole-grain bread with light mayonnaise, diced celery, and onion.

Cucumber slices with hummus dip

Day 20: 12/8

Soup with lentils, carrots, celery, and onions

Crackers made from whole grains

Day 21:

Apple slices with almond butter grilled salmon with lemon and dill served with quinoa and steamed broccoli

Dinner Meal Plan

Day 1:

Chicken breast grilled with sweet potato as well as broccoli

Fruit salad with a variety of berries

Day 2:

Brown rice with baked salmon to roasted asparagus

Salad with mixed greens, cherry tomatoes, and balsamic vinaigrette

Day 3: 26/7

Brown rice stir-fry with shrimp, bell peppers, and onions.

A fruit salad consisting of pineapple, kiwi, and mango.

Day 4: 27/7

On a piece of whole wheat bread, a grilled turkey burger includes lettuce, tomato, and avocado.

Sweet potato fries baked

Day 5: 28/7

Chili with beans and vegetables and whole grain tortilla chips

Mixed greens, cucumber, with red onion are included in a salad served as a side dish.

Day 6: 29/7

Chicken thighs baked with roasted carrots and parsnips

Quinoa salad with a vinaigrette dressing and assorted veggies

Day 7: 30/7

With roasted Brussels sprouts sweet potato mash, and grilled sirloin steak.

Mixed greens, cherry tomatoes, and cucumber make up a side salad.

Day 8: 31/7

Tofu accompanied by stir-fried veggies and brown rice.

Grapefruit, orange, and strawberries comprise a fruit salad.

Day 9: 1/8

baked cod with brown rice and roasted broccoli

Mixed greens salad dressed with balsamic vinaigrette.

Day 10: 2/8

Pork tenderloin grilled with roasted cauliflower and mashed sweet potatoes

The fruit salad consists of grapes, kiwis, and blueberries.

Day 11: 3/8

lentil soup accompanied by whole wheat bread

Mixed greens, cherry tomatoes, plus cucumber make up a side salad.

Day 12: 4/8

Chicken skewers grilled with bell peppers and onions

Quinoa salad with a vinaigrette dressing and assorted veggies

Day 13: 5/8

Salmon accompanied by roasted asparagus and quinoa.

Salad with mixed greens, cherry tomatoes, and balsamic vinaigrette

Day 14: 6/8

flank steak grilled with roasted Brussels sprouts and mashed sweet potatoes

Mixed greens, cherry tomatoes, as well as cucumber, make up a side salad.

Day 15: 7/8

Tofu accompanied by stir-fried veggies and brown rice.

A fruit salad consisting of pineapple, kiwi, and mango.

Day 16: 8/8

Chicken breast grilled with sweet potato with broccoli

Mixed greens, cherry tomatoes, and mixed cucumber make up a side salad.

Day 17: 9/8

baked cod with brown rice and roasted cauliflower

Grapefruit, orange, with strawberries comprise a fruit salad.

Day 18:

Turkey meatballs served over whole wheat spaghetti and topped with tomato sauce

Mixed greens salad dressed with balsamic vinaigrette.

Day 19:

Pork chops grilled with roasted carrots and parsnips

Quinoa salad with a vinaigrette dressing and assorted veggies

Day 20:

Brown rice stir-fry with shrimp, bell peppers, and onions.

The fruit salad consists of grapes, kiwis, and blueberries.

Day 21: 13/8

Chili with beans and vegetables and whole wheat tortilla chips

Mixed greens, cucumber, plus red onion are included in a salad served as a side dish.

21-Day Snack Meal Plan

Week 1:

Day 1: 24/7

berries on top of Greek yogurt

Putting hummus on carrots

Day 2: 25/7

Almond butter with apple slices

Chickpeas that have been roasted

Day 3: 26/7

Trail mix with string cheese and grapes (almonds, cashews, and dried cranberries)

Day 4: 27/7

Cucumber slices on top of a hard-boiled egg

Popcorn that was popped in the air

Day 5: 28/7

Pineapple and cottage cheese

Peanut butter on rice cakes

Day 6: 29/7

Tomatoes and slices of turkey

Edamame

Day 7: 30/7

Slices of orange with low-fat cheese

Homemade kale chips

Week 2:

Day 8:

Smoothie (banana, spinach, as well as almond milk) (banana, spinach, and almond milk)

Pumpkin seeds that have been roasted

Day 9:

Ricotta cheese and sliced pears

Crackers made from whole grains and hummus

Day 10:

Baby carrots with a sauce called tzatziki

Various nuts

Day 11:

Strawberry cottage cheese with low-fat cottage cheese

Roasted edamame

Day 12:

Skewers of grilled chicken and vegetables

Popcorn that was popped in the air

Day 13: 5/1

Apple slices topped with cheddar

Chickpeas that have been roasted

Day 14: 6/8

Greek yogurt with banana slices.

Sticks of vegetables with hummus

Week 3:

Day 15: 7/8

Smoothie (mixed berries, spinach, as well as almond milk) (mixed berries, spinach, and almond milk)

Peanut butter on rice cakes

Day 16:

Cherry tomatoes and low-fat string cheese

Pumpkin seeds that have been roasted

Day 17:

Low-fat cream cheese on sliced bell peppers

Trail mix (almonds, cashews, and dried cranberries)

Day 18:

Cucumber slices on top of a hard-boiled egg

Homemade kale chips

Day 19:

Cottage cheese with peach slices that is low in fat

Baby carrots with a sauce called tzatziki

Day 20:

Apple slices and turkey slices

Various nuts

Day 21: 13/8

berries on top of Greek yogurt

Crackers made from whole grains and hummus

CHAPTER FIVE

RECIPES FOR NOOM DIET FOOD LIST

Green Foods Recipes

Green Smoothie Bowl

Ingredients:

1 banana

1 cup spinach

½ of frozen mango

Frozen pineapple, half a cup

½ cup almond milk without sugar

1 tbsp of chia seeds

Directions:

Bananas, spinach, mango, pineapple, and almond milk should all be thoroughly blended.

Place the chia seeds on top of the smoothie once it has been poured into a bowl.

Dispense and savor!

Broccoli and Quinoa Salad

Ingredients:

1 broccoli head, cut into florets

1 cup cooked quinoa,

1 cup Sliced almonds

½ cup Dried cranberries

¼ cup Olive oil

2 tablespoons Apple cider vinegar

1 tablespoon of honey

To taste, add salt and pepper.

Directions:

The broccoli should be steamed until crisp-tender, then cooled.

The cooked quinoa, almond slices, dried cranberries, olive oil, apple cider vinegar, honey, salt, and pepper should all be combined in a big dish.

Toss the broccoli into the bowl when it has cooled. Enjoy.

Grilled Asparagus with Lemon and Garlic

Ingredients:

1-pound asparagus

1 lemon, juiced and zested

2 minced garlic cloves

2 tbsps of olive oil

To taste, add salt and pepper.

Directions:

Set the grill's temperature to medium-high.

The asparagus should be cut off the rough ends and put in a big bowl.

Combine the lemon juice, zest, garlic, olive oil, salt, and pepper in a separate bowl.

The marinade should be poured over the asparagus, then coated.

The asparagus should be grilled for 3–4 minutes on each side or until tender and faintly browned.

Eat and Enjoy.

Zucchini Noodles with Pesto

Ingredients:

2 substantial zucchini, spiralized

½ cup fresh basil leaves

¼ cup Pine nuts

2 Garlic cloves

¼ cup grated Parmesan cheese

¼ cup Olive oil

To taste, add salt and pepper.

Directions:

Blend the basil, pine nuts, garlic, Parmesan cheese, extra virgin olive oil, salt, and pepper in a food processor until smooth.

The zucchini noodles should be sautéed for two to three minutes at medium heat until just beginning to soften.

Toss the noodles in the pesto in the skillet and evenly distribute it.

Enjoy after serving!

Balsamic Roasted Brussels Sprouts

Ingredients:

1 pound of halved and trimmed Brussels sprouts

2 tbsp. Balsamic vinegar

1 tablespoon of olive oil

To taste, add salt and pepper.

Directions:

Set the oven's temperature to 400 °F.

Combine the balsamic vinegar, olive oil, salt, and pepper in a large bowl and stir to combine.

Brussels sprouts should be added to the bowl and mixed with the marinade.

On a baking sheet, spread the Brussels sprouts out in a single layer.

Brussels sprouts should be roasted for 20 to 25 minutes, or until they are soft and browned.

Enjoy.

Avocado and Egg Breakfast Sandwich

Ingredients:

1 English muffin with healthy grains

1 egg

sliced avocado, half

1/fourth cup of baby spinach

To taste, add salt and pepper.

Directions:

The English muffin is toasted.

Fry the egg in a small pan over medium heat until it reaches the desired doneness.

Place the baby spinach, sliced avocado, and cooked egg on one side of the English muffin before putting the sandwich together.

To taste, add salt and pepper to the food.

Serve and enjoy.

Green Bean and Mushroom Stir Fry

Ingredients:

1 pound of green beans

8 ounces of cut mushrooms

1 red bell pepper

2 garlic cloves

2 tablespoons of chopped olive oil.

2 tbsp. soy sauce

1 tablespoon of honey

To taste, add salt and pepper.

Directions:

Green beans, mushrooms, red bell pepper, and garlic should be sautéed in olive oil for 5-7 minutes over medium-high heat, or until the veggies are tender-crisp.

Mix the soy sauce, honey, salt, and pepper in a small bowl.

Toss the veggies in the skillet with the sauce after pouring it over them. Serve.

Spinach and Feta Stuffed Chicken Breasts

Ingredients:

4 skinless, boneless breasts of chicken

2 cups of infant spinach

½ cup feta cheese crumbles

1 tablespoon of olive oil

To taste, add salt and pepper.

Directions:

Turn the oven on to 375°F.

Each chicken breast should have a pocket for stuffing created by making a horizontal cut into the thickest area of the breast.

Combine the baby spinach, feta cheese, olive oil, salt, and pepper in a small bowl.

Place a piece of the spinach and feta mixture inside each chicken breast.

Bake the filled chicken breasts for 25 to 30 minutes, or until they are fully done.

Enjoy!

Kale and White Bean Soup

Ingredients:

1 tablespoon of olive oil

1 chopped onion

2 minced garlic cloves

1 bunch of chopped kale

2 rinsed and drained cans of white beans

4 cups vegetable broth

To taste, add salt and pepper.

Directions:

The onion and garlic should be softened in a big saucepan of olive oil over medium heat.

Sauté the greens in the saucepan until it has wilted.

White beans, vegetable broth, salt, and pepper should all be added to the saucepan.

The soup should simmer for 10 to 15 minutes for the flavors to come together. Enjoy.

Roasted Asparagus and Broccoli Salad

Ingredients:

1 pound of trimmed asparagus

1 pound Broccoli florets

2 tbsp. of olive oil

2 tbsp. Balsamic vinegar

1 tablespoon Dijon mustard

1 minced garlic clove

To taste, add salt and pepper.

Directions:

Set the oven to 400°F.

On a baking sheet, arrange the broccoli and asparagus florets in a single layer.

Sprinkle with salt and pepper and drizzle with olive oil.

The veggies should be baked for 15 to 20 minutes, or until they are soft and just beginning to brown.

Combine the balsamic vinegar, Dijon mustard, garlic, salt, and pepper in a small bowl.

Combine the balsamic vinaigrette with the roasted veggies.

Dispense and savor!

Zucchini Noodles with Pesto Sauce

Ingredients:

2 substantial zucchini, spiralized

½ cup of basil leaves

¼ cup Pine nuts

¼ Grated Parmesan cheese

2 minced garlic cloves

½ cup Olive oil

To taste, add salt and pepper.

Directions:

Combine the basil, Parmesan cheese, pine nuts, garlic, salt, and pepper in a food processor.

Slowly add the olive oil while the food processor is operating until the pesto is creamy and silky.

The zucchini noodles should be cooked until soft in a small amount of olive oil in a big pan over medium heat.

Combine the pesto sauce with the zucchini noodles.

Offer and savor!

Spinach and Artichoke Stuffed Portobello Mushrooms

Ingredients:

4 big Removed stems from Portobello mushrooms

2 cups of infant spinach

1 can of chopped and drained artichoke hearts

1 cup Shredded mozzarella cheese

¼ cup grated Parmesan cheese

2 minced garlic cloves

1 tablespoon of olive oil

To taste, add salt and pepper.

Directions:

Turn the oven on to 375°F.

Baby spinach and artichoke hearts should be sautéed in olive oil in a big pan over medium heat until the spinach wilts.

Stir in the garlic and cook for a further 30 seconds.

Combine the mozzarella cheese, Parmesan cheese, salt, and pepper in a small bowl.

Place the spinach and artichoke mixture into each Portobello mushroom, and then top with the cheese mixture.

For 15 to 20 minutes in the oven, the stuffed mushrooms must bake for the cheese to melt and bubble.

Serve and delight!

Green Goddess Chicken Salad

Ingredients:

1 avocado, cubed

2 cups cooked chicken

½ cup of cucumbers, chopped

½ cup of chopped celery

¼ cup freshly chopped parsley

¼ cup freshly chopped basil

2 tablespoons Greek yogurt with

2 tbsps. of olive oil

1 tablespoon lemon juice

To taste, add salt and pepper.

Directions:

Combine the cooked chicken, avocado, cucumber, celery, parsley, and basil in a large bowl.

Whisk the Greek yogurt, olive oil, lemon juice, salt, and pepper in a small bowl.

Toss the chicken salad with the dressing after pouring it over it.

Serve, and eat well!

Grilled Asparagus with Lemon Garlic Butter

Ingredients:

1 pound of trimmed asparagus

2 tbsp. of butter

1 minced garlic clove

1-tablespoon lemon juice

To taste, add salt and pepper.

Directions:

Set the grill's temperature to medium-high.

Melt the butter in a small pot.

30 seconds later, add the garlic to the pan and stir.

Add the salt, pepper, and lemon juice after turning off the stove.

The asparagus should be grilled for 3–4 minutes on each side, or until it is tender and gently browned.

Sprinkle the grilled asparagus with lemon-garlic butter.

Have fun eating!

Green Smoothie Bowl

Ingredients:

1 cup of spinach, frozen

Sliced banana, one

½ cup of pieces of frozen mango

½ cup Greek yogurt, plain

¼ cup almond milk

1 tbsp of chia seeds

Toppings include sliced bananas, kiwi, strawberries, and coconut.

Directions:

Frozen spinach, banana, mango pieces, Greek yogurt, almond milk, and chia seeds should all be combined in a blender.

Mix till creamy and smooth.

The mixture should be poured into a basin.

Sliced banana, sliced kiwi, sliced strawberries, and shredded coconut can be added to the smoothie bowl as a garnish.

Serve and have pleasure!

Yellow Foods Recipes

Turmeric Roasted Cauliflower:

Ingredients:

cauliflower head, broken up into little pieces

½ cup water

1 tbsp olive oil

1 teaspoon Turmeric

A dash of salt and pepper, to taste

Instructions:

Turn the oven temperature up to 400F (200C).

Cauliflower should be tossed in a basin with olive oil, turmeric, salt, and pepper.

Roast the cauliflower for 20–25 minutes, stirring once, until it is soft and gently browned.

Pineapple Mango Salsa:

Ingredients:

1 cup fresh pineapple, cubed

1 cup of fresh mango cubes

¼ cup of chopped red onion

3 fresh mint leaves

1 tablespoon fresh lime juice

Season to taste with salt and pepper.

Instructions:

Combine the mango, pineapple, and red onion in a bowl and toss to combine.

Blend in some fresh lime juice and season with salt and pepper to taste.

Use it as a salsa for grilled chicken or fish, or just eat it with some whole-grain tortilla chips.

Butternut Squash Soup:

Ingredients:

1 butternut squash (about a kilo), peeled and diced

1 yellow onion (about a cup's worth)

2 minced garlic cloves

½ cup water

1 tbsp olive oil

4 cups of low-sodium chicken or vegetable broth.

Nutmeg powder, half a teaspoon

To taste, with salt and pepper

Instructions:

The onion and garlic should be sautéed in olive oil in a big saucepan until they are tender and aromatic.

Toss in the butternut squash cubes and cook for another 5 to 7 minutes.

Add the broth and bring it to a boil. Simmer for 20–25 minutes, or until the butternut squash is soft.

Put in the salt, pepper, and nutmeg.

The soup may be blended with an immersion blender or transferred to a blender.

Lemon Roasted Potatoes:

Ingredients:

2 pounds yellow potatoes, diced into little pieces

¼ cup Lemon juice, freshly squeezed,

2 teaspoons Olive oil

1 tablespoon Oregano, dry

To taste, with salt and pepper

Instructions:

Set the temperature to 200 degrees Celsius (400 degrees Fahrenheit).

Combine the diced potatoes with lemon juice, olive oil, oregano, salt, and pepper in a large bowl.

Assemble the potatoes in a single layer on a baking sheet and roast for 30 to 35 minutes, turning once, until cooked and gently toasted.

Yellow Squash Casserole:

Ingredients:

2 sliced yellow squash

½ cup of chopped onion

½ cup of grated Parmesan

¼ cup breadcrumbs Mix in a bowl

¼ cup Milk, nonfat

¼ grams of olive oil

Modify with salt and pepper to taste.

Instructions:

Set the temperature to 375 degrees Fahrenheit (190 degrees C).

Olive oil should be heated over medium heat in a skillet.

Slice up some yellow squash and cut up an onion, then throw them in a pan with some olive oil and cook them till they're cooked.

Put the squash and onion in a casserole dish after cooking.

Combine the grated Parmesan, bread crumbs, and milk in a bowl. Serve over the onion and squash.

The cheese should be melted and bubbled after 20-25 minutes in the oven.

Lemon Garlic Shrimp:

Ingredients:

1 pound Peeled and deveined fresh shrimp weighing

2 tbsp. of olive oil

2 minced garlic cloves

1 tablespoon Juice of one lemon

Modify with salt and pepper to taste.

Instructions:

Warm the olive oil in a large skillet over moderate heat.

While the oil is hot, add the garlic and cook for a further minute or two until it becomes aromatic.

Sauté the raw shrimp for 2–3 minutes per side, or until they become pink and are fully cooked.

Fresh lemon juice and salt and pepper to taste should be squeezed over the shrimp.

Put on a salad or use it as a main course.

Yellow Pepper and Tomato Soup:

Ingredients:

4 cups of low-sodium chicken or vegetable broth

2 diced yellow bell peppers

1 chopped yellow onion

2 diced tomatoes

2 minced garlic cloves,

1 tbsp olive oil

To taste, with salt and pepper

Instructions:

Olive oil should be heated in a big saucepan over medium heat.

Yellow bell peppers, onion, and garlic should be diced and sautéed in the saucepan until soft.

Cook for another 5 minutes to 7 minutes after adding the chopped tomatoes.

The broth should be added and the pot brought to a boil. Simmer for 20-25 minutes at low heat.

Blend the soup with an immersion blender or in a regular blender until smooth.

Add salt and pepper to taste, then serve immediately when hot.

Here are some tasty yellow food recipes that are suitable for the Noom diet.

Spicy Yellow Curry with Tofu:

Ingredients:

1 cubed block of firm tofu

a pinch of curry powder

1 tbsp Turmeric powder

1 Tablespoon of Ground Cumin

1 Tablespoon Chili Powder

1 sliced yellow onion

2 garlic cloves, minced

1 Coconut milk in a can

2 cups Sodium-reduced vegetable broth

1 pound of chopped meat (such as bell peppers, carrots, and squash)

To taste, with salt and pepper

Instructions:

Some oil should be heated over medium heat in a big pot or wok.

Toss in the cubes of tofu and cook until they get a golden color. Take off the stove and set it aside.

Throw in some garlic and onions and cook them until the onions become transparent.

Stir in the spices (curry, turmeric, cumin, and chile) until they release their aroma.

Stir in the can of coconut milk and the veggie broth and bring to a boil.

Simmer the saucepan with the fried tofu and chopped veggies until the vegetables are cooked through.

Taste and season with salt and pepper, then serve over hot rice.

Yellow Lentil Soup:

Ingredients:

1 pound of yellow lentils

1 small onion, diced

2 minced garlic cloves

1 teaspoon of cumin powder

1 teaspoon of salt.

1 tsp. of ground coriander

1 tsp. of ground turmeric

6 cups Vegetable broth, low in sodium

Modify with salt and pepper to taste.

Instructions:

Lentils need to be soaked for at least 30 minutes in water after being washed.

Oil should be heated over medium heat in a big saucepan.

Sauté the garlic and onion until the onion is transparent.

Stir in the ground spices (cumin, coriander, and turmeric) until they release their aroma.

Rinse the lentils under cold water and add them to the cooking liquid.

Cook the vegetables in the liquid until the broth is boiling.

Turn the heat down and cook the lentils for 30–40 minutes.

Add salt and pepper to taste, then serve immediately when hot.

Yellow Zucchini Fritters:

Ingredients:

2 Grated zucchinis, yellow

½ cup all-purpose flour

¼ cup of grated Parmesan

2 Batter eggs

2 teaspoons Parsley, fresh, chopped

Just enough salt & pepper to taste

Using olive oil for frying

Instructions:

Grate the zucchini and add it to a large bowl with the flour, Parmesan cheese, eggs, parsley, salt, and pepper.

Preheat a generous amount of olive oil in a large pan over moderate heat.

Form fritters with the zucchini mixture using a spoon.

Cook the fritters for about two to three minutes on each side, or until they are golden brown and crispy.

Present hot with a salad on the side.

Red Foods Recipes

Spicy Red Pepper and Tomato Soup

Ingredients:

4 big tomatoes

1 medium onion

2 minced cloves of garlic

2 red bell peppers, sliced

1 tbsp Olive oil

4 cups of vegetable broth low in salt

1 teaspoon smoked paprika

¼ teaspoon cayenne

To taste, add salt and black pepper.

Directions:

Over medium-high heat, warm up the olive oil in a big saucepan. Cook the garlic and onion until they are transparent.

Red bell peppers as well as tomatoes should be added now and cooked for 5-7 minutes, or until softened.

Cayenne pepper, smoked paprika, and vegetable broth should be added. After bringing it to a boil, lower the heat to a simmer.

After simmering for 20 to 25 minutes, turn off the heat and let the soup to gradually cool.

Using an immersion blender or transferring the soup to a blender in stages, puree the soup until it is smooth.

To taste, add salt and black pepper to the food.

Beet and Goat Cheese Salad

Ingredients:

Chop 2 medium beets after peeling them.

4 cups of greens, mixed

¼ cup goat cheese crumbles

two teaspoons of Balsamic vinegar

1 tbsp Olive oil

To taste, add salt and black pepper.

Directions:

Set the oven to 400 °F.

Beets should be diced, then tossed with salt, pepper, and olive oil. Spread out in a single layer and roast for 20 to 25 minutes, or until tender.

Mix greens with balsamic vinegar and a dash of salt in a big bowl.

Place the mixed greens on each platter, followed by the goat cheese crumbles and roasted beets.

Grilled Shrimp Skewers with Spices

Ingredients:

1 pound of peeled and deveined big shrimp

1 red onion, diced

2 chopped red bell peppers

¼ cup olive oil

2tbps. of spicy sauce

1 tablespoon smoked paprika

To taste, add salt and black pepper.

Directions:

Heat the grill to medium-high.

Red onion, red bell peppers, and shrimp are threaded onto skewers.

Mix the olive oil, spicy sauce, smoked paprika, salt, and black pepper in a small bowl.

Grill the shrimp for 2-3 minutes on each side, or until they are pink and cooked through, after brushing them with the marinade.

Spaghetti Squash with Roasted Tomatoes and Basil

Ingredients:

1 medium spaghetti squash, seeded and cut in half.

2 cups halved cherry tomatoes

2 tablespoons of olive oil and 2 minced garlic cloves

To taste, add salt and black pepper.

¼ cup finely chopped fresh basil

Directions:

Set the oven to 400 °F.

Put the cut-side-down spaghetti squash halves on a baking sheet. Roast until soft, about 30 to 40 minutes.

Cherry tomatoes and minced garlic should be combined with olive oil, salt, and black pepper in a separate baking dish. Roast tomatoes for 15 to 20 minutes, or until they are tender and just beginning to brown.

Slice the cooked spaghetti squash into strands with a fork. Add to a large bowl and stir in chopped basil and roasted tomatoes.

Red Lentil Curry

Ingredients:

1 cup washed and drained red lentils

2 minced garlic cloves

1 red onion

1 red bell pepper.

1 tbsp Olive oil

¼ cup curry powder

¼ teaspoon cumin powder

¼ teaspoon cayenne

2 cups of vegetable broth low in salt

1 tomato diced can (14.5 ounces)

To taste, add salt and black pepper.

Directions:

Olive oil is heated over medium heat in a big saucepan. Red onion, red bell pepper, and minced garlic should all be added. Simmer for 5-7 minutes, or until veggies are tender.

Add cayenne pepper, curry powder, and ground cumin to the saucepan. Stir for one to two minutes, or until aromatic.

To the saucepan, add chopped tomatoes, vegetable broth, and red lentils. Once the sauce has thickened and the lentils are cooked, bring to a boil, then lower the heat to a simmer for 20 to 25 minutes.

To taste, add salt and black pepper to the food. For a balanced meal, serve with rice or quinoa.

Grilled Red Pepper and Chicken Kabobs

Ingredients:

1-inch chunks of each of the two red bell peppers

1 pound of cut-up, skinless, boneless chicken breasts

¼ cup Olive oil

2 teaspoons Red wine vinegar

2 minced garlic cloves

1 teaspoon Oregano, dry

To taste, add salt and black pepper.

Directions:

Heat the grill to medium-high.

Pieces of chicken and red pepper are skewered together.

Olive oil, red wine vinegar, chopped garlic, dried oregano, salt, and black pepper should all be combined in a small bowl.

The chicken should be cooked through after grilling the skewers for 5-7 minutes on each side.

Roasted Red Pepper and Cauliflower Soup

Ingredients:

2 diced red bell peppers,

1 head of cauliflower

1 medium onion

2 cloves of minced garlic

2 tablespoons of olive oil

4 cups of vegetable broth low in salt

To taste, add salt and black pepper.

Directions:

Set the oven to 400 °F.

Add olive oil, salt, and black pepper to the chopped red bell peppers, cauliflower, onion, and minced garlic. Roast for 25 to 30 minutes, or until soft and gently browned, when spread out in a single layer on a baking sheet.

Vegetable broth is added to the big saucepan with the transferred roasted veggies. Bring to a boil, then lower the heat to a simmer, cover, and cook for ten to fifteen minutes.

Blend the soup until smooth using an immersion blender or in batches in a blender.

To taste, add salt and black pepper to the food.

Tomato and Red Onion Salad

Ingredients:

2 sliced big tomatoes

1 sliced medium red onion

¼ cup red wine vinegar

two teaspoons of Olive oil

¼ cup finely minced fresh parsley

To taste, add salt and black pepper.

Directions:

Place red onion and tomato slices on a big plate.

Mix the red wine vinegar, olive oil, fresh parsley that has been finely chopped, salt, and pepper in a small bowl.

Over the tomato and red onion pieces, drizzle the dressing.

Cabbage and Carrot Slaw

Ingredients:

½ head of finely sliced red cabbage

2 grated big carrots

¼ cup of unsweetened Greek yogurt

2 teaspoons apple cider vinegar

1 teaspoon of honey

1 teaspoon Dijon mustard

To taste, add salt and black pepper.

Directions:

Red cabbage and grated carrots should be combined in a big basin.

Whisk together the plain Greek yogurt, apple cider vinegar, honey, Dijon mustard, salt, and black pepper in another bowl.

Next, coat the combination of cabbage and carrots with the dressing. Before serving, let the food cool for at least 30 minutes in the refrigerator.

Lentil and Spinach Soup

Ingredients:

1 cup red lentils

4 cups low-sodium vegetable broth

1 red bell pepper

2 carrots

2 celery stalks

1 onion, diced

2 cloves of minced garlic.

1 tomato diced can (14.5 ounces)

1 teaspoon of cumin, ground

1 paprika teaspoon

½ teaspoon cinnamon powder

Baby spinach leaves in 2 cups

To taste, add salt and black pepper.

Directions:

Lentils should be rinsed and kept aside.

Cook the veggies in a large saucepan with the onion, garlic, carrots, celery, and red bell pepper for 5 to 7 minutes, or until they are soft.

To the saucepan, add red lentils that have been washed, chopped tomatoes, and vegetable broth. Add the ground cinnamon, paprika, and cumin.

Once the soup has thickened and the lentils are cooked, bring to a boil, then decrease the heat and simmer for 20 to 25 minutes.

Stir in the young spinach leaves until they are wilted.

To taste, add salt and black pepper to the food.

Red Pepper and Feta Stuffed Chicken Breasts

Ingredients:

4 skinless, boneless breasts of chicken

2 chopped red bell peppers

¼ cup feta cheese crumbles

2 teaspoons freshly chopped parsley

To taste, add salt and black pepper.

Directions:

Turn on the 375°F oven.

Slice horizontally across the thickest section of each chicken breast, taking care not to go all the way through. This will create a pocket.

Red bell peppers, feta cheese, fresh parsley, salt, and black pepper should all be combined in a small bowl.

Place a filling of the red pepper and feta mixture inside each chicken breast.

Bake the chicken for 25 to 30 minutes in a preheated oven, or until it is well done.

Cabbage and Apple Salad

Ingredients:

½ head of finely sliced red cabbage

2 chopped apples

¼ cup chopped walnuts

¼ cup of dried cranberries

2 teaspoons apple cider vinegar

2 teaspoons Olive oil

1 teaspoon of honey

To taste, add salt and black pepper.

Directions:

Red cabbage that has been thinly sliced, apples, walnuts, and dried cranberries should all be combined in a big dish.

Apple cider vinegar, olive oil, honey, salt, and black pepper should all be combined in a different bowl.

Next, coat the combination of cabbage and apples with the dressing. Offer cold.

Red Pepper and Mushroom Frittata

Ingredients:

1 chopped red bell pepper

1 cup Sliced mushrooms

6 eggs

¼ cup of milk

¼ cup of cheddar cheese, shredded

1 tbsp Olive oil

To taste, add salt and black pepper.

Directions:

Turn on the 375°F oven.

Sliced mushrooms and red bell pepper should be sautéed in olive oil in a 10-inch oven-safe pan for about 5-7 minutes, or until the veggies are soft.

Whisk the eggs, milk, salt, and black pepper in another bowl.

After the bottom is set, cook the egg mixture over the sautéed veggies in the skillet for 3–4 minutes at medium heat.

Top the frittata with cheddar cheese that has been shredded.

After the frittata is fully cooked and the cheese has melted, place the pan in the preheated oven and bake for 10 to 15 minutes.

Red Lentil and Sweet Potato Curry

Ingredients:

1 cup red lentils

2 sweet potatoes chop after peeling them.

1 sliced onion

2 minced garlic cloves

1 tomato diced can (14.5 ounces)

1 can coconut milk (13.5 ounces)

2 teaspoons Red curry paste

1 teaspoon of cumin, ground

To taste, add salt and black pepper.

Directions:

Lentils should be rinsed and kept aside.

Cook veggies in a big saucepan with minced garlic and onion until they are soft, about 5-7 minutes.

To the saucepan, add chopped sweet potatoes, washed red lentils, diced tomatoes from a can, coconut milk from a can, red curry paste, ground cumin, salt, and black pepper.

After bringing to a boil, lower the heat, cover, and simmer for 20 to 25 minutes, or until the sweet potatoes and lentils are tender and the curry has thickened.

Serve with cooked quinoa or brown rice.

Beet and Goat Cheese Salad

Ingredients:

4 chopped, roasted medium beets

4 cups greens for a side salad

2 ounces Goat cheese crumbles

¼ cup chopped walnuts

2 teaspoons Balsamic vinegar

2 teaspoons Olive oil

1 tsp. of honey

To taste, add salt and black pepper.

Directions:

Beets can be roasted in the oven or on the stove until they are soft. Slice into bite-sized pieces after cooling.

Combine mixed salad greens, chopped roasted beets, goat cheese crumbles, and walnuts in a big bowl.

Combine the balsamic vinegar, olive oil, honey, salt, and black pepper in a separate bowl.

Toss the salad with the dressing after pouring it over it. Offer cold.

CHAPTER SIX

NOOM DIET TIPS AND TRICKS

How to stay on track with Noom Diet

Here are a few pointers to help you stick to the Noom diet's recommended food list:

Get Acquainted with the Noom Food List:

Take the time to study and comprehend the Noom food list, which classifies foods based on their caloric and nutritional richness into green, yellow, as well as red groupings.

Prepare your Meals in Advance:

Plan your meals using the Noom food list, and be sure to include an abundance of green foods, certain yellow foods, as well as a smaller number of red foods.

Keep note of Your Food Intake:

Include more green food-

Eat more green vegetables because they are healthy and low in calories. Fruits, vegetables, complete grains, and lean meats are examples of healthy foods.

Restrict Red Foods:

Red meals are heavy in calories and poor in nutrients, thus it is OK to consume them in moderation. Nonetheless, red foods should be avoided whenever feasible. Included in this category are sugary beverages, fried meals, and high-fat meats.

Be Attentive when Eating:

When you eat mindfully, you pay attention to your body's signs for when you're full and stop eating.

Request Support:

Connect with the other Noom users for assistance and accountability, and if you need assistance, contact an expert Noom coach.

How to make Healthy Food Choices

To help people, lose weight, Noom takes a behavioral approach. The color-coded food system in the Noom program is one of its most important parts. This system divides foods into 3 groups based on how many calories they have and how healthy they are. How to pick the healthiest items from the Noom Diet's food list:

Eat More Greens:

Green foods have the fewest calories and the most vitamins and minerals. Vegetables, fruits, whole grains, lean meats, and healthy fats like avocados and nuts all fall under this category. At each meal, try to fill at least half your plate with green foods.

Yellow Foods to Avoid:

The amount of calories and nutrients in yellow foods is about average. Some of these foods are whole grain bread, lean meats, dairy products, and fruits and vegetables like bananas and grapes. Even though these foods may continue to be a vital component of your diet, you should eat less of them and watch how much you eat.

Watch out for Red Foods:

Red foods have the most calories and the least amount of nutrients. These foods include packaged foods, drinks with a lot of sugar, and meats with a lot of fat. Even though it's important to eat less of these things, Noom doesn't think you should give them up completely. Instead, try to make healthier choices from these groups.

Watch out for Portions:

Noom focuses on portion size as a key part of managing your weight. Use measuring cups, cutlery, and food scales to make sure your snacks and meals are the right sizes.

Drink water:

If you drink a lot of water throughout the day, it can help you feel full and stop you from eating too much. Try to drink at least eight cups of water each day.

Pre-arrange your Meal:

Planning your meals can assist you in making healthy decisions and stop you from eating on the spot. Schedule your snacks and meals ahead of time, as well as make sure you always have healthy food on hand.

How to Plan your Meals and Snacks

Here are some suggestions for organizing your Noom Diet menus:

- ❖ How many calories do you need to consume each day? According to your age, height, weight, as well as activity level, Noom calculates a daily calorie budget for you. The amount of food you can eat every day is limited by this calorie budget.
- ❖ Noom provides a menu list from which you may select meals and snacks. Calorie density is used to divide the Noom meal list into three distinct categories. The calorie density and nutritional density of foods vary greatly, with the greenest foods having the lowest density of both and the healthiest having the greatest. You should eat more green and yellow meals and fewer red ones.

- ❖ The best way to maintain a healthy weight and eat a wide range of nutritious foods is to schedule your snacks and meals in advance. Planning your weekly meals and snacks is easy with the aid of Noom's meal planner or any similar software.
- ❖ Eat from all the food groups, and do so in a variety.
- ❖ Be careful to eat a wide range of foods out of each food category, since this will maximize the range of nutrients you take in. Green leafy veggies, a pinch of avocado (yellow food), as well as a hard-boiled egg are all examples of foods that would go well in a breakfast bowl (red food).
- ❖ Do not neglect to snack; doing so can keep you from overeating at mealtimes and keep you from feeling hungry in between meals. For a healthy snack, pick anything from the green or yellow

categories, like fresh veggies and hummus, apple and almond butter, or Greek yogurt and berries.

How to Deal with Cravings

Sticking to the Noom Diet including warding off temptations for less healthful meals can be difficult, as is the case with any eating plan or diet. On the Noom Diet, here is how to handle cravings:

Assemble your Resources:

To avoid overeating or making poor food choices, it's important to always be prepared. If you do this, you'll have a lower chance of making hasty decisions that go against your Noom objectives.

Find the Causes for Cravings:

Determine the causes of your unhealthy food desires. Can it be stress? Boredom? In a social setting? If you know what sets you off, you may develop coping mechanisms like taking a walk, phoning a buddy, or doing some deep breathing exercises.

Use the Skill of Mindful Eating:

Practice good eating habits by taking your time with each mouthful when giving in to temptation. Take note of the food's aroma, flavor, and texture. Feeling fuller for longer may help you control your food intake.

Consult the Noom Food List:

Several delicious and nutritious options that are in line with your Noom aims may be found on the Noom food list. If you're desiring something sweet, consider eating a piece of fruit or a tiny square of dark chocolate instead of reaching for a candy bar.

Don't Starve Yourself:

Starving yourself just makes you want food more. Instead, choose better options most of the time and permit yourself to enjoy your favorite meals in moderation on occasion.

CONCLUSION

One of the most well-known weight loss plans is the Noom Diet, which encourages its users to keep a food diary and make healthier eating choices. It doesn't have a stringent list of items to consume or avoid. Instead, it puts foods into the green, yellow, as well as red groups based on how many calories they have and how healthy they are.

Fruits and vegetables, which are green, have the fewest calories and the most nutrients. They must constitute the majority of your diet. Lean proteins and whole grains, which are yellow, have a little more calories per gram than other foods, but they still provide essential vitamins. Red foods, like snacks that are processed and high in calories, should be eaten less often.

The Noom Diet food list tells people to try to eat a balanced, varied diet with lots of whole, nutrient-dense foods. It also talks about how important it is to be aware and make conscious food choices instead of just following a set of rules.

This is a useful resource for those who are trying to reduce weight and enhance their health through dietary and lifestyle modifications. The Noom Diet is useful for creating long-lasting, healthful habits because it stresses the value of moderation and deliberate choice-making.

Printed in Great Britain
by Amazon

23602236R00077